THE WHOLE LIFE®

HEALTH PARTNER'S HANDBOOK

Although the health benefits in the principles expressed in this book are well known, The Whole Life's Health Partner's Handbook is neither an exercise program, diet program, nor a medical text and is not intended to replace the diagnostic expertise and medical advise of a physician. All should be certain to consult with their doctor or with a licensed health care provider before making any decisions that affect their physical health, particularly if they suffer from any medical condition or have any symptom serious enough to interfere with functioning or otherwise require treatment.

All scripture is taken from the King James Version

ISBN: 978-0-578-54264-5

Written by Joshua Vazquez, Certified Health and Wellness Coach

Edited by Hope Vazquez, Certified Health and Wellness Coach

Exterior Design by Robert Mason and Emil Baer

Interior Design by Joshua Vazquez

CONTENTS

INTRODUCTION

For every **10** people you see worldwide, **9.5** have health problems and are in need of help. What if you could do something to heal them? What if you could help without having a medical degree? What if in helping them, you could bring them to Jesus?

For the last five years, God has put a burden on my heart to heal through simple means that heal the entire person. I'm talking about things like encouraging someone to drink more water, walking with them once a week, taking them to the store and showing them how to choose produce and read food labels, showing them how to cook delicious meals in their own home—simply being a friend. By building real relationships with people and meeting their felt needs, we have built friendships that will last through eternity. As a result, people have made decisions for Christ because they found healing and wholeness in Him. Not only that, but we have seen entire churches that use this method in their outreach spring to life.

Through much prayer and lessons learned from experience, we have created this kit of resources to make it possible for *every* member, no matter what their level of knowledge and experience, to do the work Christ did. Becoming a Health Partner gives you a simple and straightforward way to connect with people on a personal level and minister to their needs. In this handbook you will learn how to use the Health Partner's Guide and the Wellness Planner, and also learn tips on how to become a proficient health partner.

Working alongside the Great Healer, you can lift burdens

and set captives free physically, mentally, emotionally, and spiritually. You, yes **you**, can spread the third angel's message and help others experience The Whole Life.

Joshua Vazquez
June 2019

Christ's method alone will give true success in reaching the people. The Saviour mingled with men as one who desired their good. He showed His sympathy for them, ministered to their needs, and won their confidence. Then He bade them, "Follow Me."

MINISTRY OF HEALING 143:3

1

WHAT IS THE NEED?

In this chapter, we are going to answer this question: what is the need? To do so, we are going to look at four major lifestyle conditions that are plaguing the world with sickness and death. Then, we will look at the top ten causes of death in the US. We will look at the prevention and the cure. Finally we will see what you and I are called to do for the saving of lives physically and spiritually.

OBESITY

Let's look at some global statistics on obesity (2016). First is the total population, then diabetes population and it's percentage:

> USA – Total Pop 324,459,463 — 129,134,866 - 39.8%
> CHINA – Total Pop 1,409,517,397 — 97,256,700 - 6.90%
> INDIA – Total Pop 1,339,180,127 — 65,619,826 - 4.90%
> BRAZIL – 209,391,872 — 41,857,656 - 20%
> MEXICO – 131,716,228 — 36,294,881 - 27.6%
> RUSSIA – 142,900,000 — 34,701,531 - 24.2%
> EGYPT – 92,000,000 — 28,192,861 - 30.6%
> TURKEY – 279,615,426 — 3,819,781 - 1.4%
> IRAN – 79,900,000 — 21,183,488 - 26.5%
> NIGERIA – 185,989,640 — 20,997,494 - 11.3%

We can clearly see there is a global obesity epidemic. The United States has the lead by far. The world population was 7,505,257,673 in 2016. The world obesity population in 2016 was over 774,000,000. Let me remind you that the estimated population of the United States was 324,459,463 in 2016 and it's obesity population (ages 20 and older) was 129,134,866.[1] These numbers mean 1 in 10 people in the world are obese. This costs the world two trillion dollars each year.[2] 1 in 7 of all obese people live in the United States and 4 in 10 adults in the United States are obese. This costs the U.S. $190.2 billion per year or nearly 21% of the annual medical spending.[3] These numbers are staggering!

DIABETES

The International Diabetes Federation reported 1 in 11 adults have diabetes (425 million) —about 90% is type II diabetes, 1 in 2 adults with diabetes are undiagnosed (212 million), and 1 in 6 births are affected by hyperglycemia.[4] The CDC reported in 2015, more than 100 million U.S. adults are now living with diabetes or prediabetes. They also reported that an estimated 1.5 million new cases of diabetes were diagnosed among people ages 18 and older.[5]

HYPERTENSION

There are over one billion people in the world with Hypertension.[6] This means that about 1 in 7 people have it. The AHA reported in 2018 that there are over 103 million Americans with hypertension.[7] Not to add insult to injury but the CDC reported in 2015 that 1 of 5 U.S. adults with high blood pressure still don't know they have it.[8] The CDC also reported in 2016 about 7 in 10 U.S. adults with high blood pressure use medications to treat the condition.[9] The cost of high blood pressure in the United States is $48.6 billion dollars each year.[8]

CANCER

In 2017 The Institute for Health Metrics and Evaluation stated that 9.6 million people are estimated to have died from the various forms of cancer throughout the world.[10] In 2016, the National Cancer Institute reported that there were an estimated 15,338,988 people living with cancer of any site in the United States. They also said, "approximately 39.3 percent of men and women will be diagnosed with cancer of any site at some point during their lifetime, based on 2014-2016 data." [11]

You might be wondering, what is causing all of this cancer? The World Cancer Research Fund (2017) estimates 20% of all cancers diagnosed in the US are caused by a combination of excess body weight, physical inactivity, excess alcohol consumption, and poor nutrition. In 2017, about 190,500 of the estimated 600,920 cancer deaths in the US will be caused by cigarette smoking, according to a recent study by American Cancer Society epidemiologists.[12]

Let's put some numbers together. Thirty one percent of cancer deaths are from cigarette smoking and another twenty percent is caused by excess body weight, physical inactivity, excess alcohol consumption, and poor nutrition. This means at least 51 percent of all diagnosed cancers come from bad lifestyle habits. Aisha Majid, Global Health Security Data Journalist, said, "These so-called 'lifestyle' conditions are a well known problem in the west. Much less understood is that they now account for the majority (53 per cent) of deaths and disabilities in the developing world – taking 31 million lives a year."[11] This means we could save the lives of 31 million people every year if we were to educate them and aid them in their lifestyle habits.

Let's shift our focus to the US. It's top three killers account for 51 percent of mortality. They are:

1. Heart Disease
2. Cancer
3. Chronic Lower Respiratory Disease

In fact, when you look at the top ten killers in the United

States you begin to see a stunning correlation. These are the top ten killers in the United States and their preventions according to the National Vital Statistics Reports and the CDC:[14]

1. HEART DISEASE
Control your blood pressure, keep your cholesterol and triglyceride levels under control, stay at a healthy weight eat a healthy diet, get regular exercise, manage stress, manage diabetes, limit alcohol, don't smoke, and make sure that you get enough sleep.

2. CANCER
Don't use tobacco, protect yourself from the sun, maintain a healthy weight and be physically active, eat plenty of fruits and vegetables, avoid obesity, limit processed meats, drink alcohol in moderation, get immunized, avoid risky behaviors, and get regular medical care.

3. ACCIDENTS
Unintentional poisonings (number one is drug overdose), unintentional falling, and unintentional vehicle accidents.

4. CHRONIC LOWER RESPIRATORY DISEASE
Do not smoke, exposure to second hand smoke, vapors, gases, dust, or fumes, practice good hygiene, practice a healthy lifestyle, and avoid sick people.

5. STROKE
Exercising more, eating better, and maintaining a healthy weight, controlling your blood pressure, stopping smoking, and drinking only in moderation, managing your blood sugar level and diabetes, and treating any underlying heart defects or diseases.

6. ALZHEIMER'S DISEASE
Exercising and remaining physically active throughout your life, eating a diet filled with fruits, vegetables, healthy fats, and reduced sugar, treating and monitoring any other chronic diseases you have, and keeping your brain active with stimulating tasks like conversa-

tion, puzzles, and reading.

7. DIABETES
Reaching and maintaining a healthy weight, exercising for at least 30 minutes, five days a week, eating a healthy diet with plenty of fruits, vegetables, whole grains, and lean proteins, and having regular blood sugar checks if you have a family history of the disease.

8. INFLUENZA AND PNEUMONIA
Washing hands frequently, especially after blowing nose, going to the bathroom, diapering, and before eating or preparing foods, quitting smoking - tobacco damages the lungs and reduces the ability to fight off infection, smokers have been found to be at a higher risk of getting pneumonia, and good health habits - a healthy diet, rest, regular exercise, etc. - help prevent viruses and respiratory illnesses.

9. KIDNEY DISEASE
Follow instructions on OTC medications, especially when using non-prescription pain relievers, avoid excessive intake of alcohol, maintain a healthy weight, quit smoking, and manage medical conditions with the help of a doctor or health care professional.

10. SUICIDE
Depression, psychosis, impulse while drunk or high, they're crying out for help, and don't know how else to get it, they have a philosophical desire to die, they've made a mistake.

Reading through these you begin to see a pattern: getting regular exercise, eating a healthy diet, staying at a healthy weight, practicing good hygiene, making sure you get enough sleep, eliminating alcohol, and not smoking seem to be the best preventative measures. All ten killers are caused by one or more of these poor lifestyle choices.

31 million people in the world die because of poor lifestyle

habits. In the US, 51 percent die from the same causes. 53 percent of the world's deaths could be stopped. Do you know someone who has died or is fighting one of these diseases today? What if you could save them? Would you do it? Would you invest the time, energy, and effort to save them? I can only imagine that your answer is, "YES!"

"**My people** are destroyed for lack of knowledge:" Hosea 4:6. In this text, God is referring to His people in the church. Our membership is allowing their health to fall through the cracks. However, this message is not for Seventh-Day Adventists alone: "And I heard another voice from heaven, saying, Come out of her, **my people**, that ye be not partakers of her sins, and that ye receive not of her plagues." Revelation 18:4. The word that is used here is the Greek word "plege" - "a public calamity, heavy affliction." Does 31 million people sound like a public calamity or heavy affliction? In my humble opinion, absolutely.

What is the solution?

"…If thou wilt diligently hearken to the voice of the LORD thy God, and wilt do that which is right in his sight, and wilt give ear to his commandments, and keep all his statutes, I will put none of these diseases upon thee, which I have brought upon the Egyptians: for I am the LORD that healeth thee." Exodus 15:26

What Commandments do you think God is talking about in this verse? He is talking about the Ten Commandments. Let's see what the Spirit of Prophecy says about the commandments:

"Our first duty, one which we owe to God, to ourselves, and to our fellow men, is to obey the laws of God. These include the laws of health." Counsel on Health, 24.2

Looking back at Exodus 15:26 it used the word "statues." In the Greek, that is the word "choq" - "statute, ordinance, limit, something prescribed, due." God told Israel, if they kept His "commandments" (laws of health) and His "statues" (prescriptions), He would "put none of these diseases upon them, which I have brought upon the Egyptians:". If you think how I think, you are probably wondering, what were the diseases the Egyptians were having? "A 2011 study of 52 mummies in the Egyptian Museum in Cairo showed that almost half had clogged arteries, the kind of condition that can lead to a heart attack or stroke."[15] Not only were their arteries clogged, inducing heart attacks and strokes, they also had diabetes, obesity, and cancer. Could it be that God has laid out a specific prescription for us to follow? After all, He did say in the same verse, "for I am the LORD that healeth thee."

God's people needed healing. Don't forget there was a mixed multitude that came out of Egypt. Not only that, but the Israelites were eating the same things that the Egyptians were eating. They were addicted to the flesh pots and lifestyle of Egypt. What prescriptions did God give them? "Pure air, sunlight, abstemiousness, rest, exercise, proper diet, the use of water, trust in divine power—these are the true remedies." —Counsel on Health, 90.2. We are going to see this is exactly the prescription God gave His people as soon as they crossed the Red Sea.

The following passage is from Exodus 15:27-16:4, 22, 23. I have pointed out the "true remedies" in the "[ ]'s":

"And they came to Elim, where were twelve wells of water [water], and threescore and ten palm trees: and they encamped there by the waters. And they took their journey [exercise, fresh air, and sunshine] from Elim, and all the congregation of the children of Israel came unto the wilderness of Sin, which is between Elim and Sinai, on the fifteenth day of the second month after their departing out of the land of Egypt. And the whole congregation of the children of Israel murmured against Moses and Aaron in the wilderness: And the children of Israel said unto them, Would to God we had died by the hand of the LORD in the land of Egypt, when we sat by the flesh pots, and when we did eat bread to the full; for ye have brought us forth into this wilderness, to kill this whole assembly with hunger. Then said the LORD unto Moses, Behold, I will rain bread [nutrition] from heaven for you; and the people shall go out and gather a certain rate [temperance] every day, that I may prove them [trust in divine power], whether they will walk in my law, or no. And it came to pass, that on the sixth day they gathered twice as much bread, two omers for one man: and all the rulers of the congregation came and told Moses. And he said unto them, This is that which the LORD hath said, To morrow is the rest [rest] of the holy sabbath unto the LORD: bake that which ye will bake to day, and seethe that ye will seethe; and that which remaineth over lay up for you to be kept until the morning."

Who followed the children of Israel in the wilderness? "Moreover, brethren, I would not that ye should be ignorant, how that all our fathers were under the cloud, and all passed through the sea; And were all baptized unto Moses in the cloud and in the sea; And did all eat the same spiritual meat; And did all drink the same spiritual drink: for they drank of that spiritual Rock that followed them: and that Rock was Christ." 1 Corinthians 10:1-4. Jesus followed them in the wilderness. What were the remedies Jesus used to heal His people that were addicted to the lifestyle of the Egyptians? "Pure air, sunlight, abstemiousness, rest, exercise, proper diet, the use of water, trust in divine power..." Counsel on Health, 90.2

HEALTH PARTNERING AND THE THIRD ANGEL'S MESSAGE—

Did you know that the first five prophets in the Bible are repeated in Revelation 14? Who was the first prophet the Bible gives reference to? Enoch. What was special about Enoch? He walked and He never saw death. Revelation 14:1-5 talks about who? The 144,000 who walk with God and never see death.

Let's look now at the first angel's message, "And I saw another angel fly in the midst of heaven, having the everlasting gospel to preach unto them that dwell on the earth, and to every nation, and kindred, and tongue, and people, Saying with a loud voice, Fear God, and give glory to him; for the hour of his judgment is come: and worship him that made heaven, and earth, and the sea, and the fountains of waters." Revelation 14:6, 7. Who was the type of the first angel? "And spared not the old world, but saved Noah the eighth person, a preacher of righteousness, bringing in the flood upon the world of the ungodly;" 2 Peter 2:5 What type of message is it that Noah was preaching? A worldwide message of judgment and that there is safety in the sanctuary (the ark). The same as the first angel.

Let's look at the second angel's message, "And there followed another angel, saying, Babylon is fallen, is fallen, that great city, because she made all nations drink of the wine of the wrath of her fornication." Revelation 14:8. What is one of the major problems with Babylon? One of the major problems with Babylon was image worship. Who else in the Bible was called out of Babylon because of image worship? "And Terah took Abram his son, and Lot the son of Haran his son's son, and Sarai his daughter in law, his son Abram's wife; and they went forth with them from Ur of the Chaldees, to go into the land of Canaan; and they came unto Haran, and dwelt there." "And Joshua said unto all the people, Thus saith the LORD God of Israel, Your fathers dwelt on the other side of the flood in old time, even Terah, the father of Abraham, and the father of Nachor: and they served other gods." Genesis 11:31;Joshua 24:2, 3, 14

God called Abram out of Babylon because his family was nearly consumed with image worship. Abram is the type of the second angel. Was Abram called out of Babylon to serve God in sincerity and in truth? Yes, he was. This is what the second angel's message calls us to do.

Let's move on to the third angel's message. "And the third angel followed them, saying with a loud voice, If any man worship the beast and his image, and receive his mark in his forehead, or in his hand, The same shall drink of the wine of the wrath of God, which is poured out without mixture into the cup of his indignation; and he shall be tormented with fire and brimstone in the presence of the holy angels, and in the presence of the Lamb: And the smoke of their torment ascendeth up for ever and ever: and they have no rest day nor night, who worship the beast and his image, and whosoever receiveth the mark of his name. Here is the patience of the saints: here are they that keep the commandments of God, and the faith of Jesus." Revelation 14:9-12.

What laws are included in the Ten Commandments? The Laws of Health are included in the Ten Commandments. Is the third angel's message the final message that is to prepare God's people to enter into the promised land? Yes, it is. Who is the type of the third angel? "And the LORD said, I have surely seen the affliction of my people which are in Egypt, and have heard their cry by reason of their taskmasters; for I know their sorrows; And I am come down to deliver them out of the hand of the Egyptians, and to bring them up out of that land unto a good land and a large, unto a land flowing with milk and honey; Come now therefore, and I will send thee unto Pharaoh, that thou mayest bring forth my people the children of Israel out of Egypt." Exodus 3:7, 8, 10. Was Moses the final messenger to prepare God's people to enter into the promised land? Yes, he was! Moses is a type of the third angel.

After God delivered Israel from Egypt, what did He give them? "And said, If thou wilt diligently hearken to the voice of the LORD thy God, and wilt do that which is right in his sight, and wilt give ear to his commandments [laws of health], and keep all his statutes [prescriptions], I will put none of these diseases upon thee, which I have brought upon the Egyptians: for I am the LORD that healeth thee." "Pure air, sunlight, abstemiousness, rest, exercise, proper diet, the use of water, trust in divine power—these are the true remedies." Genesis 15:26; Counsels on Health, 90.2 Hold that thought. We will come back to it momentarily.

Who was it that took God's people into the promised land? "But charge Joshua, and encourage him, and strengthen him: for he shall go over before this people, and he shall cause them to inherit the land which thou shalt see." Deuteronomy 3:28. Joshua took God's people into the promised land. Who is Joshua a type of? Joshua is a type of Jesus. It is Jesus that will lead us into the promised land. What happens after the third angel's message? Jesus takes the righteous to the promised land.

Let's take this a step further. Who prepared the way for Jesus' first advent? John the Baptist. What was John the Baptist famous for? John the Baptist was famous for baptisms. Do you know who isn't as famous for baptisms but might have more baptisms than John? "Moreover, brethren, I would not that ye should be ignorant, how that all our fathers were under the cloud, and all passed through the sea; And were all baptized unto Moses in the cloud and in the sea;" 1 Corinthians 10:1, 2.

Moses was also a type of John the Baptist. He prepared the way for Joshua as did John the Baptist for Jesus. What was John the Baptist's Message? "Prepare ye the way of the Lord, make His paths straight". Didn't Moses' message prepare God's people for Jesus' coming? "How", you ask? Moses' message was "Prepare ye the way of the Lord" in reference to them building the sanctuary. After all, the Shakina Glory is the visible presence of Jesus. "And let them make me a sanctuary; that I may dwell among them…And the Word was made flesh and dwelt among us" Exodus 25:8; John 1:14

What is the purpose of the sanctuary? It's purpose is to show us the great sacrifice that Jesus made for us and the atonement He is making for us right now in the Heavenly sanctuary. Why did Jesus give them the remedies before He had them build the sanctuary?

"Those who place so much food upon the stomach, and thus load down nature, could not appreciate the truth should they hear it dwelt upon. They could not arouse the benumbed sensibilities of the brain to realize the value of the **atonement** and the **great sacrifice** that has been made for fallen man. It is impossible for such to appreciate the great, the precious, and the exceedingly rich reward that is in reserve for the faithful overcomers." Counsels on Health, 158.2

Jesus gave them the remedies before they built the sanctuary because it would be impossible for them to see the value in it otherwise.

Let's pull it all together now. The condition of the world's health is beyond saddening. 31 million people are dying every year that should not. The minds of hundreds of millions of people are so beclouded that they could not appreciate the truth should they hear it dwelt upon. However, God has risen up a people who are called to give every nation, kindred, tongue, and people life, and that they might have it more abundantly. A work that is so relevant and so needed. So much so that sister White said this:

"We have come to a time when **every member** of the church should take hold of medical missionary work." Testimonies for the Church, vol. 7, page 62.1

Jesus gave us an example in the wilderness between Egypt and the promised land. In the next chapter we will see that Jesus used the exact same method when He became flesh. We will also learn about the incredible science behind the method Jesus used in the wilderness, when He came, and what He wants to use through you in your community.

What is the need?

"The world needs today what it needed nineteen hundred years ago—a revelation of Christ. A great work of reform is demanded, and it is only through the grace of Christ that the work of restoration, physical, mental, and spiritual, can be accomplished." The Ministry of Healing, 142, 143 (1905).

2

WHY HEALTH PARTNERING?

What I hope to convey to you in this chapter is the great need for health partners in the Seventh-Day Adventist Church. I believe that EVERY member should be a health partner. In this chapter, we will answer four questions that, I hope, will cause you to see the great need for this work in the world and in our churches. Here are the four questions:

1. What was Christ's method?
2. How does Christ's method relate to health partnering?
3. How do we use health partnering in ministry?
4. How will it affect you and God's church?

1. WHAT WAS CHRIST'S METHOD?

We will not spend too much time on this question because the next chapter will build on the answer to this question. Let's begin by looking at the words of Jesus in Luke 17:19, "And he said unto him, Arise, go thy way: thy faith hath made thee whole." Here Jesus tells the leper he is now "whole." What does it mean to be whole? The Greek word used here for "whole" is "'sozo", which means to save from physical and spiritual destruction.

'Sozo is the same word that is used in Matthew 9:22, "But Jesus turned him about, and when he saw her, he said, Daughter, be of good comfort; thy faith hath made thee whole. And the woman was made whole from that hour." This passage gives us an amazing insight about Christ's method. It says that she was "made whole from that hour." This gives us the answer to question number one, "what was Christ's method?" Christ's method was a simultaneous healing of the physical and the spiritual. One good question we should ask ourselves is this: Has Christ's method changed over the years? Not at all. Therefore, according to the quote on the inside cover, if we want "true success," our method should facilitate a simultaneous healing of the physical and the spiritual.

2. HOW DOES CHRIST'S METHOD RELATE TO HEALTH PARTNERING?

Let's begin to answer this question by reading John 17:18. "As thou hast sent me into the world, even so have I also sent them into the world." Here, Jesus tells the Father what He has commissioned us to do—the same work He did. "Christ's work is to be our example…He preached the gospel and healed the sick." "During His ministry, Jesus devoted more time to healing the sick than to preaching." "The first and chief object of the gospel and all that pertains to it is to seek and to save that which is lost. The ministry of the gospel, whether by the minister or the physician, is to reach out to man a helping hand wherever it is needed. It is to minister to the sick and suffering physically as well as to the sin-sick soul." Testimonies for the Church vol 9, pg. 31.1; Ministry of Healing pg. 19.4; A Call to Medical Evangelsim 43.4

In light of "'sozo", can you picture Jesus healing and preaching at the same time? Imagine, that as He tenderly spoke of the unending love and grace of His Father, He touched those who were deemed untouchable, restoring them wholly. "His miracles testified to the truth of His words, that He came not to destroy, but to save." Ministry of Healing pg. 19.4. What a sight it must have been! What an amazing day it will be when the Holy Spirit is poured out and we will be able to heal the multitudes' physical and spiritual maladies by a single touch.

How can we fulfill the prayer of Jesus by healing the physical and the spiritual? The Holy Spirit showed me an amazing principle when I was studying this out in Romans 12:2. "And be not conformed to this world: but be ye transformed by the renewing of your mind, that ye may prove what is that good, and acceptable, and perfect, will of God." Transformation happens by the renewing of the mind. Therefore, the renewing of the mind causes transformation. Paul then states the purpose of transformation, "that ye may prove." What does that word "prove" mean? The word "prove" means "to recognize as genuine after examination, to approve, deem worthy." The apostle tells us that when we are transformed, by the renewing of the mind, we now have the ability to deem worthy "what is that good, and acceptable, and perfect, will of God." Here is the equation: **Renewing of the mind = transformation = deeming worthy the will of God.**

This concept may be a paradigm shift for you as it was for me. Does the mind really have to be physically renewed for us to appreciate spiritual truths?

"It is impossible for men and women, while under the power of sinful, health-destroying, brain-enervating habits, to appreciate sacred truth... Every violation of principle in eating and drinking blunts the preceptive faculties, making it impossible for them to appreciate or place the right value upon eternal things... It is impossible for an intemperate man to be a Christian, for his higher powers are brought into slavery to the passions." Counsels on Health pg. 21.2, 38.2, 36.1 [If you would like more quotes on this concept, search "it is impossible" in the book Counsels on Health.]

How do bad lifestyle habits physically effect the brain? The four brain scans on the right show the effect of blood flow on a brain that is under the influence of alcohol (second), cannabis (third), and finally caffeine and nicotine.[1] It may be surprising to you, but the most impaired

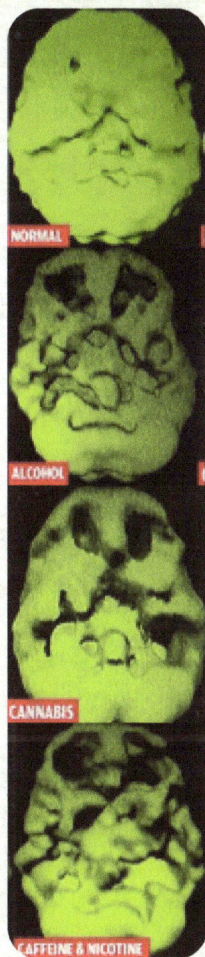

NORMAL

ALCOHOL

CANNABIS

CAFFEINE & NICOTINE

brain is the one under the effects of caffeine and nicotine. Can you think of anyone who drinks coffee, energy drinks, caffeinated sodas, or tea? What about people who are using any of the different forms of nicotine?

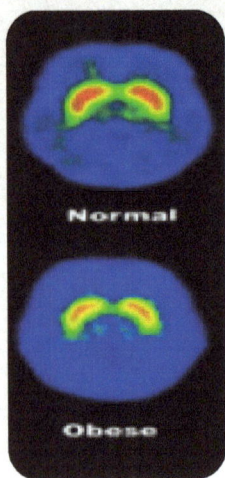

The two brain scans on the left show significantly less dopamine (happy hormone) receptors due to obesity. Something found in people who are addicted to drugs.[2] Does it make more sense now that it is impossible for humans to appreciate truth without a physical transformation happening first?

How can a health partner renew the mind? We do it by helping people follow the laws of health. The first law (we will only look at a few) is water. Drinking water is easy for most and you will see why you will begin with this law when we get to chapter five. Look at what Dr. Corinne Allen, founder of the Advanced Learning and Development Institute said, "Brain cells need two times more energy than other cells in the body. Water provides this energy more effectively than any other substance."

Amazing things begin to happen when your new friend begins to drink water! Did Jesus get people to drink water? Let's see what Mark 9:41 says. "For whosoever shall give you a cup of water to drink in my name, because ye belong to Christ, verily I say unto you, he shall not lose his reward." Jesus wants us to give people water when they need it. Most people are not drinking enough.

What about sleep? Read what Michael Thorpy, director of the Sleep-Wake Disorders Center at Montefiore Health System and professor of clinical neurology at Albert Einstein College of Medicine said, "The lymphatic system of the brain opens up at night, and removes toxins while we're asleep."

Notice that the toxins of the brain are released at night— while we are asleep. Sleep at night is best if we want toxins to be released from the lymphatic system in the brain. How much sleep is necessary? Eight and a half hours for adults is best. Dr. Eve Van Cauter states that children need about ten hours, those aged twelve to twenty-one require about nine hours. For adults, research indicates that those who sleep more than ten hours may have negative side effects.

Research shows that sleep deprivation can seriously effect our brain. Studies show that if you go without sleep for eighteen hours straight, you suffer from a level of impairment that is equal to having a blood alcohol content of 0.05 percent.[3-5] If you go without sleep for twenty-four hours, the impairment is equal to having a 0.10% blood alcohol content, and you are seven times more likely to have an accident.[5-6] Look at this brain scan from Penn State University of someone doing mathematical problems while rested, then sleep-deprived:

EFFECT OF SLEEP DEPRIVATION ON BRAIN ACTIVATION WHILE PERFORMING MATHEMATICAL TASKS.

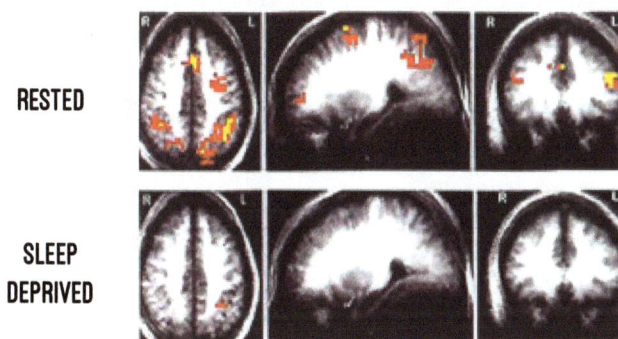

RESTED

SLEEP DEPRIVED

The sleep-deprived brain is nearly inactive compared to the brain that has had ample sleep. Jesus invites all, "Come unto me, all ye that labour and are heavy laden, and I will give you rest." Matthew 11:28. Health partners take on the same work. They invite others to get the right amount of rest at the appropriate times. As your new friends in the community begin to find rest, their mind will be renewed.

Health partners encourage people to get adequate amounts of sunshine. Does being outside in the sunshine help with the renewing of mind? Let's see what Professor Allen Butterfield of the University of Kentucky says, "Adequate vitamin D serum levels are necessary to prevent free radical damage in the brain and subsequent deleterious consequences."

"Free radicals" are unstable atoms that cause damage to the body through oxidization, contributing to aging and disease. However, sunshine gives the body the vitamin D it needs to prevent free radical damage to the brain. The less damage to the brain, the better the function of the whole system.

Did Jesus encourage people to get sunshine? Let's see what it says in Malachi 4:2. "But unto you that fear my name shall the Sun of righteousness arise with healing in his wings; and ye shall go forth, and grow up as calves of the stall." Being in the rays of the Sun brings healing.

There is one more thing I want to cover that health partners encourage people to do—get active. Most commonly, the most people will be able to do is walk. Walking is the most important thing that you will do with people. You might be questioning the previous statement. You are probably thinking, "No, getting them to trust in Divine power is the most important." You have a good point. I will, however, "stick to my guns" on this and will explain more a little later.

How does walking help with the renewing of the mind? Look at the brain scan/research done by Dr. Chuck Hillman of the University of Illinois:

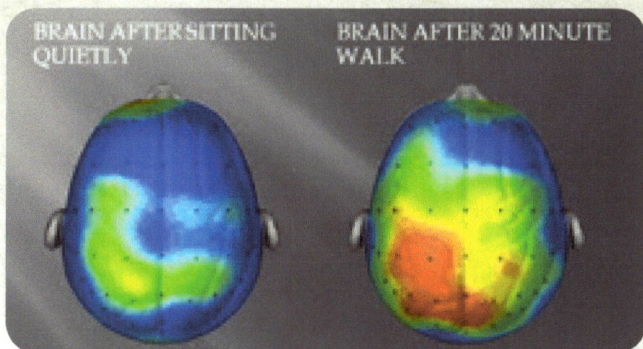

BRAIN AFTER SITTING QUIETLY

BRAIN AFTER 20 MINUTE WALK

Notice how much the activity of the brain increases after a twenty minute walk— just a walk. There was no crazy sprinting or a 45 mile bike ride uphill, just a twenty minute walk.

If there was ever someone that got people to walk, it was Jesus. "During His ministry Jesus lived to a great degree an outdoor life. His journeys from place to place were made on foot, and much of His teaching was given in the open air." "they followed him on foot out of the cities." Counsels on Health pg. 162.2.; Matthew 14:13

We have seen a few of the laws of health and how they help with the renewing of the mind. We have also seen how health partnering facilitates Christ's method in a practical way and the close relationship they have with one another.

3. HOW DO WE USE HEALTH PARTNERING IN MINISTRY?

"Health reform, wisely treated, will prove an entering wedge where the truth may follow with marked success." Selected Messages Book 3, pg. 285.3. Health reform can be an entering wedge. In fact, this is the wedge Jesus used most.

I have learned something about an "entering wedge" through my experience as a wellness coach. An "entering wedge" not only opens the door, but, when wisely treated, it keeps the door open. This is what makes Christ's method so successful. Even if the person doesn't make the spiritual step right away, a friendship is made which allows opportunity for future cultivation.

Think about the great harvest Jesus reaped during His life—there wasn't one. The harvest came after His death, resurrection, and pentecost. Why? Because His method left an "entering wedge" that kept the doors of their hearts cracked. This allowed the Holy Spirit to swing the door open wide as a mighty rushing wind, and the early rain watered the seeds Jesus planted through His healing and preaching. Now, please don't get discouraged and think that there won't be any harvest until the latter rain. People are already coming to Jesus because of this method. Christ is constantly drawing people to Him and securing their souls in the kingdom.

I told you earlier I would talk about why I believe exercising with people, particularly walking, is the most important of the health laws. Here is why: when you walk with someone, you are doing it because you see a need, you have sympathy, and you desire their good, right? And when you walk and talk with people, what begins to build? A relationship begins to build. As you build a relationship with someone, do they begin to tell you things they normally wouldn't? Most of the time, yes. Why is that? They do so because they begin to have confidence in you. I would now like us to look at the quote from Ministry of Healing pg. 143.3:

"Christ's method alone will give true success in reaching the people. The Savior mingled with the men as one who desired their good. He showed His sympathy for them, ministered to their needs, and won their confidence. Then He bade them, 'Follow Me.'"

This is exactly what happens when you walk with someone. Could saving a soul be that easy? "We do not understand the matter of salvation. It is just as simple as ABC. But we don't understand it." Faith and Works pg. 64.3.

Could it be that someone could be saved because they are regularly walking with someone who cares about them? Are we not saved because we regularly walk with Someone who cares about us? "And Enoch walked with God: and he was not; for God took him." Genesis 5:24

Enoch and God walked together so much and their relationship was so strong that God could not bear to live without Enoch and He took him home. The word here for "took" also means "to lead." If you lead someone, the person you are leading follows you, right? Couldn't we read this verse as…"And Enoch walked with God: and he was not; for God bade him, follow me."

By working to renew the mind you have placed the wedge for the Holy Spirit to perform a mighty work. So what exactly does it mean to renew the mind? I believe renewing the mind, in a physical sense, means to restore the frontal lobe of the brain. The frontal lobe is your "heart." It is where you decide whether you are going to do good or evil. It is were you will recieve the seal of God or the mark of the beast. By renewing this part of the brain you help people see spiritual things more clearly. They will begin to make better decisions in every aspect of their life. They will not only see that the Advent message is true but they will apprecate it and see the value in following it.

So, to answer question number three, we use health partnering as an entering wedge to facilitate a simultaneous transformation of the physical and the spiritual.

4. HOW WILL HEALTH PARTNERING AFFECT YOU AND GOD'S CHURCH?

I'd like to take you to a little church in Spirit Lake, Idaho. A city with a population of just over 2,000. In 2015, there was an attendance of about 40 on Sabbath. Through the blessing of the Holy Spirit this church began to do health partnering in the community which led to relationships, friendships, and baptisms.

This church began to see and admire the beauty in Christ's method. They began to help people clean up their yards and they planted a garden to give fresh food to their new friends in the community. They helped people move, clean their houses, shoveled snow from roofs and driveways. As they united to go out of their way to help others, there began to form a bond between the members that grew deeper and deeper. This work began to foster an atmosphere of love that caused an explosion in this church.

This little church that once had an attendance of 40 became the fastest growing church in the North Pacific Union (per-capita) and pushed 90-100 present on Sabbath, in just two years. There are church members that had left the church who have now come back, people from the community who have found the truth and better health, youth that went into the waters of baptism, and families that drive an hour and a half to join them every Sabbath.

Friends, imagine the true success we would have if we renewed the mind before we displayed our precious pearls of truth. Imagine if the minds of those we are studying the Bible with were clear enough to hear the gentle whisperings of the Holy Spirit. What if we were known as the church who heals the community? What if you were known as the Christian that heals and preaches? You know, I have actually met a Man who did this. The Bible says He had healing in His wings and the multitudes flocked from all over for "'sozo."

His spiritual impact on the world is still felt over two thousand years later and He spent most of His time healing —not preaching. What spiritual impact could we have on the world if we spent most of our time healing rather than preaching?

He is calling us all to follow in His footsteps today. How will health partnering affect you and God's church? Both will experience Jesus in His fullness.

3

CHRIST'S METHOD - CASTING THE VISION

In this chapter, we are going to see some of the same material we saw in chapter two. This repetition is not only to reinforce the concept of health partnering, but also to show how it is a practical application of Christ's method. Health partnering prioritizes personal relationships and meeting felt needs while intentionally looking for opportunities to share the Gospel. This is lacking in the current evangelistic model, which has become impersonal and focuses on sharing a knowledge of the truth without demonstrating it. I humbly believe that in order to experience the true success spoken of in Ministry of Healing pg. 143, we need to align our evangelistic priorities with Christ's method.

Many churches use event-based evangelism. Events are a wonderful opportunity to meet new people and generate interest in what the church is doing. However, when the majority of outreach is done through events, there is little time or opportunity to connect on a more personal level. The events require a large expenditure of time and energy to prepare for, yet come and go very quickly. If a greater emphasis were placed on personal evangelism, these events would be more productive and effective. To illustrate, let's use the example of a church hosting a healthy cooking class. A visitor comes because they had some level of interest in improving their health. After experiencing the class, they are excited to start using some of what they learned. Or maybe they feel a little overwhelmed but still want to make changes. At the end of the class, someone announces that health partners are available that will assist them in their health journey and help them make goals that work for them. They will even help them learn to use recipes like the ones demonstrated, right in their own kitchen! The visitor signs up because this is just what they needed. It is a relevant answer to a felt need. Now we have a direct connection to that visitor, and a church member will be connecting with them on a one-on-one basis, developing a friendship with them. I believe that every event should have a follow-up that will allow church members to build relationships between events, and health partnering is a natural and friendly way to do it.

This is what Jesus' method is all about. He wanted to connect with people on a personal level so He could tell them about His Father. He calls us to do the same today. If we reduced the number of events and spent more time in personal, one-on-one interaction, meeting felt needs, building relationships, and telling people about our Father, I think we would be surprised at the results.

Let's read from the chapter entitled "The Work of the Disciples" in Ministry of Healing pg. 143.3. "Christ's method alone will give true success in reaching the people. The Savior mingled with the men as one who desired their good. He showed His sympathy for them, ministered to their needs, and won their confidence. Then He bade them, 'Follow Me.'" If you break this down, you could see that Jesus spent most of His time one-on-one with people meeting their felt needs. "During His ministry, Jesus devoted more time to healing the sick than to preaching. His miracles testified to the truth of His words, that He came not to destroy, but to save." — Ministry of Healing pg. 19.4

I find it interesting that "His miracles testified to the truth of His words." Why weren't the words of the Word Himself enough to convert people? "Though I speak with the tongues of men and of angels, and have not charity, I am become as sounding brass, or a tinkling cymbal. And though I have the gift of prophecy, and understand all mysteries, and all knowledge; and though I have all faith, so that I could remove mountains, and have not charity, I am nothing. And though I bestow all my goods to feed the poor, and though I give my body to be burned, and have not charity, it profiteth me nothing. Charity suffereth long, and is kind; charity envieth not; charity vaunteth not itself, is not puffed up, Doth not behave itself unseemly, seeketh not her own, is not easily provoked, thinketh no evil; Rejoiceth not in iniquity, but rejoiceth in the truth; Beareth all things, believeth all things, hopeth all things, endureth all things. Charity never faileth:" —1 Corinthians 13:1

The words of the Word would have been empty without the miracles to go along with it. I like to call it "Christ's method of charity." Charity suffers long, is kind, believes all things, hopes all things, endures all things, and it never fails.

It is by mingling as one who desires their good, showing sympathy, and ministering to their needs, on a personal level, that we win their confidence. Then will they clearly hear the Shepherd's voice.

Now let's do some reviewing from chapter two. What was Christ's method? "But Jesus turned him about, and when he saw her, he said, Daughter, be of good comfort; thy faith hath made thee whole. And the woman was made whole from that hour." —Matthew 9:22 The healing that Jesus did was 'sozo. 'Sozo means to save from physical and spiritual destruction. When did Jesus save people from their physical and spiritual destruction? "From that hour" or simultaneously. Christ's method is a simultaneous healing of the physical and the spiritual.

How are we supposed to work to fulfill the great commission? "As thou hast sent me into the world, even so have I also sent them into the world." "Christ's work is to be our example...He preached the gospel and healed the sick." —John 17:18; 9T 31.1

BUILDING THE BRIDGE —

What is the purpose of health partnering? "And be not conformed to this world: but be ye transformed by the renewing of your mind, that ye may prove what is that good, and acceptable, and perfect, will of God." —Romans 12:2 The purpose of a wellness coach is to renew the mind to what God intends it to do—know his will.

How is it that health partners accomplish this? "Pure air, sunlight, abstemiousness, rest, exercise, proper diet, the use of water, trust in divine power—these are the true remedies." —Counsels on Health pg. 90.2.

Water is the first law that you want to begin to implement. Due to the length of time you will spend in your first session, it is the perfect fit. It also helps the body get ready for activity.

The next law you will introduce is activity. This is the most important, so it needs to be next in line. You want to begin your friendship with them as soon as possible. Walking is the best way to do it. This is a great way to show Christ's method of charity. By walking with them you are mingling as one who desires their good, showing sympathy, ministering to their needs, and winning their confidence. I cannot stress enough the importance of walking WITH them. Don't over schedule yourself to where you can't walk with them. This will greatly hinder your effectiveness.

Nutrition is the next law to introduce. Healthy and tasty meals are what they need to be taught. Don't forget to meet them where they are! Just because you have been eating like an Adventist your whole life doesn't mean it is easy. Unhealthy food is addicting. Please, be mindful.

"The more produce you eat, the better off your memory will be. Folic acid, a B vitamin found in peas, broccoli, spinach, artichokes, beets and oranges, appears to be particularly helpful." —Joy Bauer, RD. It is fascinating to me that eating more produce helps your memory. Remember that word "memory."

Next teach them about the importance of fresh air.

"Researchers at Harvard looked at the decision making abilities of 24 people, who were exposed to different indoor working conditions over six days. The findings, published in the journal Environmental Health Perspectives, showed those with higher levels of pollutants were less able.

"Researchers at Harvard looked at the decision making abilities of 24 people, who were exposed to different indoor working conditions over six days. The findings, published in the journal Environmental Health Perspectives, showed those with higher levels of pollutants were less able.

Participants scored an average 61 percent higher while working in buildings with low pollution levels, compared to days working in a conventional building. They were tested on everything from basic tasks to crisis response and information seeking.

'These results suggest even modest improvements to indoor environmental quality may have a profound impact on the decision making performance of workers.'" — Dr Joseph Allen, director of the healthy buildings program at the Harvard Centre for Health and the Global Environment.

"Decision making"…I think you should remember that one too.

Next, share with them the benefits of being out in the sunshine. "Adequate vitamin D serum levels are necessary to prevent free radical damage in brain and subsequent deleterious consequences." — Prof. Allan Butterfield, University of Kentucky

Tell them about the wonderful results they will get when they experience better rest, that their performance in many things will increase and they will be more able, physically and mentally. .

Teach them temperance. Lovingly and gently each them to stay away from cigarettes, alcohol, caffeinated beverages, and all things that are bad for them.

The image below shows how "nicotine from a cigarette attaches to the a4ß2*-nACh receptors in the brain, it displaces a radio labeled tracer (red and yellow indicate high levels of the tracer, green indicates intermediate levels, and blue indicates low levels). The nicotine from three puffs displaced 75 percent of the tracer from study participants' receptors, and the nicotine from three cigarettes, nearly all."[1]

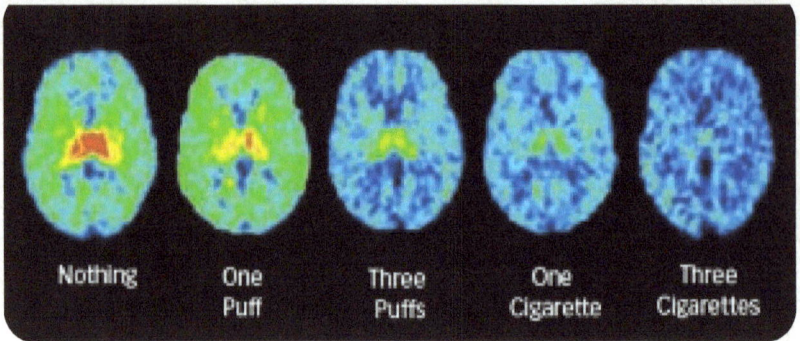

The scans below show the true affect of wine on someone who drinks one to two glasses of wine each day (right). This is the amount that was allegedly healthy and encouraged for you to consume. This study was done by the AMEN Clinic and published on May 17, 2016.

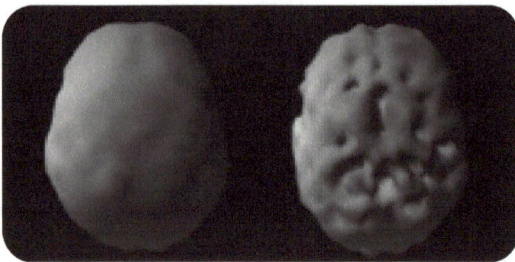

Teach them the importance of hygiene. How doing simple things like brushing and flossing teeth, bathing, regular laundry, and washing their hands can actually save their life. Not just physically but socially as well. Teach them the importance of food safety and of a neat and orderly environment.

There is a principle that is necessary for you to grasp as a Christian and as a Christian health partner. It is found in the following two verses: "Be ye not unequally yoked together with unbelievers: for what fellowship hath righteousness with unrighteousness? and what communion hath light with darkness?" "This then is the message which we have heard of him, and declare unto you, that God is light, and in him is no darkness at all." —2 Corinthians 6:14; 1 John 1:5

The principle is this, where there is light, there can be no darkness. As the Holy Spirit begins to share light in their life and renew their mind, there is no more room in their life for the bad.

For example, I was coaching a woman that would drink 16 cups of coffee each day and didn't drink water. She had a phobia of tap water. Growing up in WWII Germany, there were many reasons you didn't drink from the tap. To overcome this obstacle, she set a goal of drinking 3 four-ounce cups of water each day for a week. Well, that week she ended up drinking about 5 or so tall glasses of water. Guess what happened to her coffee intake? It began to drop because the water (light) pushed out the coffee (darkness).

So often we want to strip people from all of their bad habits at once. The principle of adding light is a great way to work with the Holy Spirit and not instead of the Holy Spirit. Please remember, don't get upset and don't give up if they don't make the changes that you wish they were making. God is working on them. When they are struggling, it is a great opportunity for you to share your testimony of how temperance has helped you in your life. Don't forget Christ's method of charity: It suffers long, is kind, believes all things, hopes all things, endures all things, and it never fails.

OPENING THE BRIDGE —

The laws of health that we have just covered pave the way for where we want to lead them— trust in Jesus. Let's see what you have just allowed the Holy Spirit do through you as a wellness coach. Wait…"memory" and "decision making"…got it.

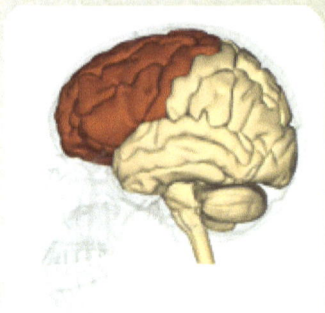

The red part on the brain to the right is the frontal lobe. The frontal lobe controls the following functions: memory, decision making, judgment, impulse control, discerning good and evil, and your motor functions. Do these six functions sound important in the Christian walk? Are we not sealed in our frontal lobe?

All of the natural laws assist and improve all of these functions. These laws of health help build the bridge (frontal lobe) which is the main part of the brain activated when we communicate with God! Notice what happens to the blood flow in the brain scan below from Dr. Andrew Newberg, the physiological focus shifts to the frontal lobe.[2] Amazing!

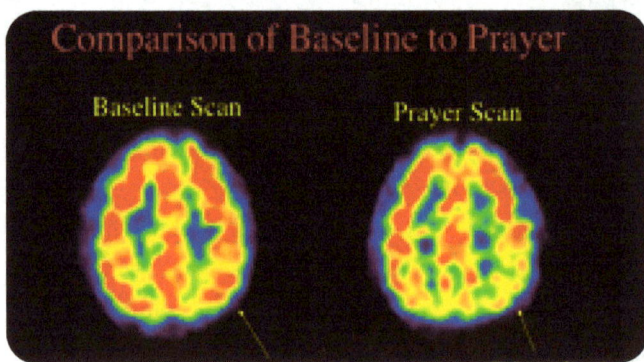

Comparison of Baseline to Prayer

Baseline Scan   Prayer Scan

Are you ready to work with Jesus and like Jesus? Are you connected to Him? "I am the vine, ye are the branches: He that abideth in me, and I in him, the same bringeth forth much fruit: for without me ye can do nothing." John 15:5. In order to work like Jesus you must know who He is and have a constant connection with Him through the indwelling of the Holy Spirit. Would you like to move forward in the full power of the Holy Spirit and show the world what Jesus is like?

4

THE FUNDAMENTALS OF HEALTH PARTNERING

If I were to define health partnering, I would say it is the easiest way for anyone to win a soul to Jesus. Not everyone can be on the radio, television, preach, or be a pastor. Not everyone is a nurse or a physician. However, anyone can be a health partner.

WHAT KIND OF DEGREE DO I NEED? —

One of the many questions I get is, "how much medical training do I need to be a health partner?" The answer is, not much at all. What is great about this program is that the 8 Laws of Health DVD does most of the teaching for you. However, "A practical knowledge of the science of human life is necessary in order to glorify God in our bodies. It is therefore of the highest importance that among the studies selected for childhood, physiology should occupy the first place." —Counsels on Health pg. 38.1. Please allow me to add, if you don't have a practical knowledge of human physiology, it's never too late to get some!

As of 2018, there are no official standardizations in the field of wellness coaching. There are institutions that do give certifications for it, such as Eden Valley Institute (where I attended) and Weimar's HEALTH Program (where my wife attended). Another great resource is the Rocky Mountain Conference's Health Ministries Director, Rick Mautz. There is a seven-video series of him instructing a class at Eden Valley. The web address is: http://www.rmcsda.org/health-ministries-coaching-copy-07-23-2015-12-24-am.

The difference between health partners and wellness coaches is the amount of training received. Wellness coaching training varies anywhere from 6 months to a year. Whereas a health partner training can be done on a weekend. I also want to make it clear that The Whole Life Health Partner Training or materials does not give you any type of certification. It teaches you, what is being called in the Adventist circle, how to be a "Health Partner."

As a health partner you are simply being a support and a friend, encouraging and guiding people to reach their own health goals. Furthermore, you are not there to diagnose, treat, or undermind their physician —it is illegal for you to do any such thing. It is good to encourage those you are partnered with to communicate with their doctor as they are making progress in healthy living, as it may require medication adjustments by their physician.

What Does a Health Partner Do? —

Essentially, a health partner facilitates and guides their friend's path to wellness. This program is to be entirely personalized to each individual. Therefore, it is key that the partner guides their friend to make their own goals. The partner is to never make a goal for the person they are coaching unless permission is granted. Setting up a goal is achieved through active listening and asking open-ended questions.

A Competent Health Partner —

There are two main skills that a competent Health Partner has—active listening and the ability to ask open-ended questions. If you can do these two things well, you will be a very successful partner.

To be a good, active listener, you will need to do the following things:

➢ Mirror the other person's emotions. If the person is sad, be sympathetic. If they are excited about something, be excited with them.

- ➤ Repeat their question before you answer. Repeating their question not only shows them that you are listening and that you care, but it also helps you to ensure you understand the question so you can answer the question correctly.
- ➤ Give reassuring gestures when they are talking, i.e. nodding your head, eye contact, one word reassurances, etc.
- ➤ DON'T BUT IN!!! There is nothing worse than someone trying to finish your sentences for you. Especially if they get it wrong. Let the person fully express themselves. Wait until they are done speaking, and then talk if needed. You are there to listen and help them. It's not the other way around.

Open-ended questions are questions that can not be answered with "Yes," "No," "Maybe," or any other one-word response. Open-ended questions usually lead into other questions. This technique is great when you can see a change someone needs to make. You can use open-ended questions to lead the person to discover the change that needs to be made.

SILENCE IS GOLDEN —

Don't be afraid of silence after asking a question. It may be a bit awkward at first, but silence after a question is a good thing. It means they are thinking and trying to find the answer. This is a great tool to learn if you are giving Bible studies also. If the silence last for a really long time, ask them if they understood the question. If not, try to rephrase the question and let them think on it.

PUTTING THEM INTO PRACTICE —

The wonderful thing about active listening and asking open-ended questions is that you can practice these skills everywhere. Practice asking open-ended questions at the grocery store, bank, post office, church, with your spouse, children, boyfriend, girlfriend, any and all family, friends, coworkers, and random people you run in to.

SAMPLE QUESTIONS —

- ➢ How would you like to see yourself by the end of the twelfth session?
- ➢ What does ideal wellness look like for you personally?
- ➢ What are some things you want to be doing when you have achieved your ideal wellness?
- ➢ What are some obstacles that are keeping you from achieving your wellness vision or have kept you from achieving better health?
- ➢ What are some strategies you can use to over come those obstacles?
- ➢ What motivates you in life?
- ➢ What do you value most in your life?

These questions can open up a lot of someone's life. Not only that, it also helps you build a relationship, gives you more information to be able to link them with other church members, and allows you to know how you can pray for them. Please keep this information confidential.

HEALTH PARTNERING DO'S AND DON'TS —

DO'S:
- ➢ Renew your rapport and trust at the beginning of each session.
- ➢ Always ask permission for prayer or for offering suggestions.
- ➢ Ask your friend how they are feeling and use active listening.
- ➢ Explore strengths from past to build confidence.
- ➢ Discuss the gap between now and the desired vision.
- ➢ Assist with realistic small steps in setting goals to build confidence.
- ➢ Challenge your friend to aim high if you think they can.
- ➢ Empathize with friends' feelings and needs, accept them where they are.
- ➢ Explore their best experiences, values, and deep wishes.

- ➤ Keep an upbeat, positive attitude at all times, even with resistance.
- ➤ Praise your friends of their efforts and focus on the positive changes.
- ➤ Balance over-praising and under-praising based on your friend's needs.
- ➤ Show appreciation for the challenges of making and maintaining changes.
- ➤ Revisit motivators when needed.
- ➤ Use humor to lighten the mood.
- ➤ Remember important days that they have mentioned: birthdays, anniversary, doctors visits, etc.
- ➤ Change failures into "learning opportunities" or "life lessons."
- ➤ Be supportive and encourage family and friend support.
- ➤ Speak the truth in love to build self esteem and hope.
- ➤ Stay current in health and wellness news.
- ➤ Recognize when to refer to specialist.
- ➤ Affirm their good work and your desire to walk with them in their journey.
- ➤ Get regular input regarding what is or is not working in partnering sessions.

DON'TS:
- ➤ Interrupt or cut off your friends while they are speaking.
- ➤ Talk too much
- ➤ Play psychotherapist
- ➤ Wear the expert hat, unless your friend gives you permission requesting such assistance.
- ➤ Assume you understand what your friend is saying —ask and clarify.
- ➤ Impose your goals on your friend. They need to make their own goals.
- ➤ Push your friend beyond their capabilities.
- ➤ Become impatient with a lack of change.
- ➤ Focus on yourself or your issues during sessions.
- ➤ Allow your friend to dwell on topics outside of your partnering scope.

THE PROGRAM —

The initial commitment is twelve sessions— one session each week, for twelve weeks. Many people will need longer to fulfill their physical and spiritual needs. This is why I let them know, in the beginning, at the end of the twelfth session we can reassess to see if they would like to continue the partnership. Please note that ideally the program is twelve weeks if they don't miss a session. However, if they miss a week the program is now thirteen weeks. If they miss two weeks during the program, the program now becomes fourteen weeks, etc. There must be twelve sessions to complete the program and receive the completion certificate.

The programs is like a staircase. The final step on the staircase is where they want to be— their perfect picture of health. It is basically the finish line. However, like all staircases, there are some steps that need to be taken before you get to the top step. The small steps that help them reach the top step are the weekly goals.

Each week a new goal will be set based on the 8 Laws video by Life & Health network. On week one they will set their wellness vision and their water goal for that week. On the second week they will set the goal for exercise and adjust the water goal higher if they achieved it, lower if it was too difficult, or keep it the same if they almost achieved it yet it is still challenging enough to keep. Each week a new goal is added and the previous week is adjusted. See the Week-by-Week Session Outline on page 48.

5

ʏᴏᴜʀ ꜰɪʀꜱᴛ ᴘᴀʀᴛɴᴇʀɪɴɢ ꜱᴇꜱꜱɪᴏɴ

For this chapter you will need The Whole Life: Health Partner's Guide.

Your first coaching session will take one and a half to two hours. The majority of your time will be helping them set up pages 8 and 9 of their Wellness Planner. You will do this by having your Health Partner's Guide open to page 24. Please, turn there now. As you can see there are three different colored sections. Each color corresponds with each section. Page 25 is the page your new friend sees in the Wellness Planner. The blue section, on page 24, gives you instructions on how to help them fill out the "Wellness Vision" section on page 25.

Now we are going to look at each section individually and talk about each one. We will begin with the "Wellness Vision" section which is on page 24 of the Health Partner's Guide.

ꜱᴇᴛᴛɪɴɢ ᴜᴘ ᴛʜᴇ ᴡᴇʟʟɴᴇꜱꜱ ᴠɪꜱɪᴏɴ —

The Wellness Vision is who they want to be and what they want to be doing. One common vision that I get is, "I want to have the same size waist I had in high school." That is a perfectly acceptable vision. However, the length of time that will take can vary extensively depending on how far they have gotten from their high school waist size. A wellness vision can be a twelve week vision or it could be a five year vision. It all depends on their vision.

How do you help your friend discover what their vision is? It is through active listening and open-ended questions. Keep in mind that the more you practice asking open-ended questions, the quicker you will begin to develop your own style and proficiency. Here are some sample questions to help you:

- What does ideal wellness look like for you personally?
- What are some things that you would like to be doing regularly that are difficult for you to do now?
- How would you like to see yourself at the end of the 12 week program?
- What are some things you want to be doing when you have achieved your ideal wellness?

Remember that silence is golden after you ask a question. Give time for their wheels to turn and the lightbulb will turn on. There is another rule that I am quite a stickler about. Don't let them say "I will try…" "When I can…" or "I would like to…" They need to write, "I will" as part of their goal. Words can make or break a person. We want to be as affirmative and positive as possible.

Once they have their wellness vision figured out have them write it down in the "Wellness Vision" section on page 8 of the Wellness Planner. See the example below:

WELLNESS VISION

Your Wellness Vision is who you ultimately want to be and what you want to be doing when you reach the top of your staircase. Once you reach these goals, all you will have to do is maintain the habits that have become your lifestyle!

MY WELLNESS VISION IS

I will weigh 150 pounds and be diabetes free!

I will be able to play with my grandchilden without getting tired so quickly.

IDENTIFYING OBSTACLES —

Identifying their obstacles is going to be a very useful tool for you. This will show you what they have tried in the past and why it didn't work. This will help you see if they are motivated or not so motivated. It could be that they have certain medical conditions that obstruct their progress. One common obstacle for people that have been overweight for a long time are bad knees.

They will discover obstacles the same way they discovered their wellness vision—through their health partner who is actively listening and asking them open-ended questions. They do not need to write "I will" when writing their obstacles. See the example of common obstacles people face.

OBSTACLES
What events, circumstances, or habits are standing in the way of reaching your Wellness Vision?

MY OBSTACLES ARE

I do not prioritize myself and I am busy taking care of
other people. I make excuses. I am lazy.

HURDLING OBSTACLES —

The next phase, after you help them discover their obstacle, is to ask them what they can do to overcome these obstacles. If they don't come up with anything quickly, ask them some open-ended questions to help them figure it out. It may be helpful to find out what their strengths are and use them to overcome their weaknesses. Don't forget to have them write "I will…"

STRATEGIES
What are some new methods or habits that will help you overcome your obstacles?

MY STRATEGIES TO OVERCOME MY OBSTACLES ARE

I will begin to prioritize myself and learn to say "no."
I will stop making excuses and being lazy because I realize
they are only making me miss out on things that are
truly important to me.

FINDING MOTIVATORS —

Things that motivate people are usually things that are of value to them i.e. God, children, spouse, and even pets. These valuables are great motivators that help people strengthen their commitment to the task at hand. If you hold these motivators in the mind it will help them stay on track.

MOTIVATORS
What will motivate you to stay on track? Is it longevity with your family and friends, losing a few pant sizes, fighting disease, or something else?

MY MOTIVATORS ARE

My family, not being sick anymore, having more energy, living long enough to see my great grand children.

SETTING UP A SUPPORT SYSTEM —

You are probably going to be their number one supporter. Furthermore, this is a great place in the session to find out some good information about them— primarily, if they attend a church. Ask them if they have any people that will support them on their new journey to wellness. Then ask them if they belong to any organizations/clubs i.e. a church or a gym.

SUPPORT SYSTEM
Are there any people, organizations, or clubs that you are affiliated with that will support you in your wellness journey?

MY SUPPORT SYSTEM

People: My husband, my daughter

Organizations/Clubs: None

This is where I decide if, at the end of the session, if should ask them if they want prayer. If they go to church, 99.99 percent of the time they will be open to it. If they don't go to church, it is probably a very good idea to hold off until you begin to build a relationship and know more about them. I say probably a good idea because you must always be willing to change things up according to the command of the Holy Spirit.

WEEKLY SESSIONS —

Each session has it's own section in the Wellness Planner. It has key points from the 8 Laws video for you to review after the video is played. There are also tips for success that you should go over as well. More impor antly are the questions that are asked on these pages.

They are asked to list some things they learned in the video clip that affect them personally. Make sure you have them fill this out at the end of each video! They might need some help. So, use the information that they have told you or some information that you have gathered, through observation, to help them figure it out. You also want to make sure that you talk to them about what they write down each time. This will get them used to you asking them about what they write down. The purpose of this is to open up conversation when you get to the eighth law —trust in divine power. By doing this regularly you can eventually find out where they are spiritually and not make them feel like you are being pushy.

Turn to page 28 in the Health Partner's Guide to see the step-by-step instructions in this area.

SETTING WEEKLY GOALS —

Weekly Goals are what will help your friend reach their wellness vision. They are the make or break factor in the program.

They will help your friend stay on track and get excited about their progress. This is where your help will be needed to make sure they don't set their goals too high or too low. Having a failing grade every week is discouraging. On the other hand, setting goals that are too easy doesn't give a sense of accomplishment. Worried about helping them gauge whether they set a good goal? Ask the Holy Spirit. He will help you!

They will set the weekly goal after you watch a short segment from the 8 laws video. Use the information that is in the video as a guide for the goals. Use the same techniques that you used to set the wellness vision, namely, active listening and open-ended questions. Make sure that the goals are SMART. SMART: Specific, Measurable, Attainable, Relevant, and Time Sensitive.

WHAT IS YOUR WATER GOAL FOR THIS WEEK?

I will drink 50 oz of water each day.

I will buy a water bottle and use it.

LOGGING PROGRESS —

Throughout the week they will need to log what they have accomplished each day. There are examples in the Wellness Planner and the Health Partner's Guide for each of the goals they need to log. There are also Daily Meal Logs and Thankfulness Logs beginning on pages 59 and 69. Just in case your friend missed some sessions there are a three sets of extra logs on pages 78-92.

Daily Water Log

Example of Daily Water Log

60 oz.	65 oz.	65 oz.	65 oz.	70 oz.	70 oz.	75 oz.

WEEK-BY-WEEK SESSION OUTLINE—

Here is an outline of what you need to do during each appointment. The pages correspond with the Wellness Planner:

SESSION 1:
1. Watch the 8 Laws overview video (pause the video).
2. Set up the wellness vision, explore obstacles and strategies to overcome the obstacles, find motivators, and set up a support system.
3. Push play on the video to watch the video on water.
4. Review key points from the video, answer the questions, and review the tips for success on pages 10 and 11.
5. Set up the water goal for the first week on page 31.

SESSION 2:
1. Go for a walk to gauge the ability to exercise.
2. Review the water log on page 31 to see how they met their goal and adjust goals as needed.
3. Watch the video on exercise.
4. Review key points from the video, answer the questions, and review the tips for success on pages 12 and 13.
5. Set up an exercise goal for the week on page 32.

SESSION 3:
1. Go for a walk.
2. Review the water and activity log to see how they met their goals and adjust goals as needed.
3. Adjust water and exercise goals as needed.
4. Watch video on nutrition.
5. Review key points from the video, answer the questions, and review the tips for success on pages 14 and 15.
6. Set up nutrition goal of the week on page 33.

SESSION 4:

1. Go for a walk.
2. Review logs from the past week to see how they met their goals and adjust goals as needed.
3. Watch video on fresh air.
4. Review key points from the video, answer the questions, and review the tips for success on pages 16 and 17.
5. Set up a fresh air goal for the week.

SESSION 5:

1. Go for a walk.
2. Review logs from the past week to see how they met their goals and adjust goals as needed.
3. Watch video on sunshine.
4. Review key points from the video, answer the questions, and review the tips for success on pages 18 and 19.
5. Set up a sunshine goal.

SESSION 6:

1. Go for a walk.
2. Review logs from the past week to see how they met their goals and adjust goals as needed.
3. Watch video on rest.
4. Review key points from the video, answer the questions, and review the tips for success on pages 20 and 21.
5. Set up a rest goal.

SESSION 7:

1. Go for a walk.
2. Review logs from the past week to see how they met their goals and adjust goals as needed.
3. Watch video on temperance.
4. Review key points from the video, answer the questions, and review the tips for success on pages 22 and 23.
5. Set up a temperance goal.

SESSION 8:

1. Go for a walk.
2. Review logs from the past week to see how they met their goals and adjust goals as needed.
3. Watch video on trust in divine power.
4. Review key points from the video, answer the questions, and review the tips for success on pages 24 and 25.
5. Set up prayer goal for that week if they are open to it.

SESSION 9:

1. Go for a walk.
2. Review logs from the past week to see how they met their goals and adjust goals as needed.
3. Read pages 26-28 about hygiene and complete page 29.
4. Set up a hygiene goal.

SESSION 10:

1. Go for a walk.
2. Review all logs to see how they met their goals.
3. Adjust all previous goals as needed.

SESSION 11:

1. Go for a walk.
2. Review all logs to see how they met their goals.
3. Adjust all previous goals as needed.

SESSION 12:

1. Go for a walk.
2. Review all logs to see how they met their goals.
3. Adjust all previous goals as needed.
4. Reassess to see if they want to continue the program or terminate.

6

HOW TO MAKE NEW FRIENDS

MEETING FRIENDS AT THE DOOR —

"Now Jacob's well was there. Jesus therefore, being wearied with his journey, sat thus on the well: and it was about the sixth hour. There cometh a woman of Samaria to draw water." —John 3:6, 7

Jesus went to the well because He knew He had a divine appointment with the woman. Why was she there? She was there because she had a need. Was the way she was fulfilling her need working for her? No, it was not. Jesus knew of her need, went to where she was going to be, and met her there. Then He introduced what He had to offer.

In your case, your are offering a health partnership program. In order to be able to secure appointments, there are four key things you must do at the door when introducing the program after giving the Community Health Survey:

➤ You must be clear.
➤ You must be short.
➤ You must be to the point.
➤ You must believe in the program.

Notice how Jesus tells her that her habits were sustaining her but not completing her. Then He showed her what He had to offer in John 4:13, 14:

"Jesus answered and said unto her, Whosoever drinketh of this water shall thirst again: But whosoever drinketh of the water that I shall give him shall never thirst; but the water that I shall give him shall be in him a well of water springing up into everlasting life."

Did Jesus believe in what He had to offer? He believed without question. He also knew the main "selling" points. Here are your four main selling points:

1. I never tell you what to do— the program is completely personalized.
2. No crazy diets.
3. No equipment needed.
4. Only $30 for 12 weeks ($2.50 a session) and guaranteed results.

If you make sure they understand these four selling points, you have done your best.

THE PURPOSE OF A SURVEY —

The purpose of a survey is to facilitate further inquiry of the answers given by the person receiving the survey. This will help you get more information which you can use to show them their need for the program. The more information you can get in relation to their health, the better chance of getting them to sign up. You have done a good job at giving a survey when you get them to sign up without completing all of the questions on the survey.

HOW TO GO —

"After these things the Lord appointed other seventy also, and sent them two and two before his face into every city and place, whither he himself would come." —Luke 10:1

Going two by two is how we are instructed to go. This gives

great advantage because while one is giving the survey, the other is praying inconspicuously. Usually when the person giving the survey is "stuck," their companion is prompted by the Holy Spirit with the right words to say. This makes a powerful team.

You should dress to fit the area you are going to knock in. Don't dress up too much in a lower income area. Business casual should work just fine for most places. If you are going into an area of high-income, perhaps slacks, dress shirt, and tie for men and a professional skirt and blouse for women would be appropriate. Dress modestly and simply.

Prayer and doing your best is going to be your only guarantee for any success in every part of this ministry. Ask for the Holy Spirit to go with you and before you to clear the way and show them their need. Ask Him to give you the right words to say and the power to say them.

"And Jesus came and spake unto them, saying, All power is given unto me in heaven and in earth. Go ye therefore, and teach all nations, baptizing them in the name of the Father, and of the Son, and of the Holy Ghost: Teaching them to observe all things whatsoever I have commanded you: and, lo, I am with you alway, even unto the end of the world. Amen." —Matthew 28:18-20

EVENTS AND CHURCH ACTIVITIES —

Other ways to make new friends is at events like evangelistic meetings, health expos, AMEN Clinics, cooking classes, depression recovery classes, week of prayers, Sabbath services, fair booths, etc.

FRIENDS, FAMILY, AND CHURCH MEMBERS —

A great place to start is with those you know already. This will help you gain expierence and confidence as a health partner.

Not only that, but you will begin healing those you love most. What a wonderful way to live —helping others experience The Whole Life.

7

WHAT YOU'VE BEEN WAITING FOR

I can imagine that by now you are wondering when I'm going to tell you how health partnering leads to Bible studies. So far you have seen that health partnering in principle is the primary means of delivering the third angel's message. You've seen that this is the method Jesus used during His life on earth and even before His incarnation. But exactly how do we go from helping people become healthier to opening the Word with them and ultimately leading them to Christ?

I'm going to share some tips from my experience that I pray will be helpful to you.

But first, I want to re-emphasize that physical and spiritual healing go hand-in-hand. Jesus never healed someone physically without also healing them spiritually. It was a healing of the whole person. You must realize that health partnering is not a bait-and-hook program to lure people into Bible studies. The entire journey of health partnering brings about a spiritual transformation. As you're helping people become healthier, you're preparing the mind to appreciate truth as the frontal lobe clears. You're developing a relationship of trust that makes people more comfortable opening up and talking about spiritual things. And as they begin to feel better, they will get excited about learning what else you have to share. They have had an experience just as the people Jesus healed did, and they will tell the world about it.

WHERE'S THE COOKIE CUTTER? —

Everyone is different. Each person has a different personality and character and they are in a different place spiritually. If I were to tell you that there is an approach that worked for every person, every time, I'd be lying to you. I have worked with atheists, agnostics, Christians, substance-abusers, nice people, mean people, motivated people, and unmotivated people. I can say there isn't a specific phrase or question to make the transition.

THE PATIENCE OF A SAINT —

As much as we'd like to expect a certain time-frame to get to the Bible studies, some people take a long time to get to the point where you can approach them about spiritual things. For example, it took over a year for one lady I worked with before I was even able to pray with her! I waited patiently and never tried to offer prayer before she was ready. Six months after that first prayer, she was baptized. Another lady I worked with took three years of meeting off and on before she was baptized. Others are ready and I'm praying with them early on.

RED, YELLOW, AND GREEN —

One thing I have learned is to pay attention to how people respond when I drop little seeds. A good time to drop seeds is on your walks. You are in the open air, in nature, and you are not across the table staring at them in the face (which can make it awkward for them). If they respond positively, you have a green light to plant more seeds soon. Plant your seeds tactfully. Don't try to plant too many at once—it could backfire. Remember the words of Jesus: "I have yet many things to say unto you, but ye cannot bear them now." Always proceed with prayer and let the Holy Spirit guide you.

If their response isn't a definite green light, but they aren't completely closed, consider that a yellow light and proceed with caution. I personally would wait a session or two before I try again. By waiting, you can avoid seeming pushy and they will be less likely to put up walls.

If they respond negatively or reject the seed, consider that a red light. This is when you do not want to plant any seeds for a long time. In this situation, it is best to not get offended or seem upset that you have been rejected. Simply smile and let them know you are here to help them where they are comfortable being helped.

Let me give you examples of these three scenarios. Let's say you are coaching a woman named Sally. You are on session seven and she tells you and your companion that she didn't meet her goals this week because she had a really hard week at work. You then say, "Oh no, what happened?" She tells you how a coworker spread rumors about her and everyone was treating her poorly. At the end of the session you say something like this, "Sally, I feel terrible that you had to deal with that this past week. Would it be okay if we pray with you about this situation, that it can be resolved and your reputation cleared?" If she says something like, "that would be great" or "I would appreciate that," in a favorable tone, you have a green light. This may mean she is open to regular prayer after each session. If someone gives me the green light for prayer, I make sure I pray with them each future session.

If she says something along the lines of, "Umm...I guess so" or "Suuure," in a reluctant tone, I would still pray with her but would be very careful next time. She has given you a yellow light.

If she says, "I'd rather not" or "I'm good," you have received a red light. When I get a red light for prayer, I do not pray with them. I smile and reassure them that I am here to help them, and that prayer is part of the program but they are in control of what goals they wish to set or not to set. It will be important to remember this when you get to session eight. In session eight, everyone will have the opportunity to be prayed with. Make sure you don't unnecessarily cause them to feel uncomfortable if they reject prayer or anything spiritual.

WHAT IF I GET A RED LIGHT? —

So you have just been given a red light. This can be discouraging. However, not all is lost. Yes, all red lights mean "Stop," but some mean, "Not right now." Do you remember the lady that it took me a year to pray with? I got the red light the first time I met her at her door while doing the health survey. She said, "You're not going to preach to me are you?" I said, "I won't mention God if you don't mention God." We made a deal to stay at the red light until she changed it to green.

This is why the program is a minimum of twelve sessions and we are willing to work with them for as long as it takes. There are some people that don't want to continue the coaching after the twelve sessions but they were willing for me to meet with them once a week just to walk with them. This is my way of keeping in contact and it gives me the opportunity to drop some seeds every now and then. Others really enjoy the sessions and want to continue them.

HERE IS THE COOKIE CUTTER —

In conclusion, the most important thing to realize is that you need to let the Holy Spirit be in control—always. When you listen to His promptings, you will do the right thing. There are times when He prompts me to break all of the "rules." There are other times when I was going to break the "rules" because I thought it was the right thing to do, and He kept me from doing it. He knows what, where, how, and when to say what you need to say. It is His work and He knows what He is doing. You are only His agent. Be patient. Don't give up on them. Jesus hasn't given up on you.

WORK CITED

CHAPTER 1

1. Health, United States, 2017, table 53, CDC

2. Dobbs R., Sawers C., Thompson F., Manyika J., Woetzel J.R., Child P., McKenna S., Spatharou A. *Overcoming Obesity: An Initial Economic Analysis.* McKinsey Global Institute; Jakarta, Indonesia: 2014

3. Cawley J, Meyerhoefer C. *The medical care costs of obesity: an instrumental variables approach.* Journal of Health Economics. 31(1):219-230. 2012.

4. IDF, Diabetes Atlas 8th Edition, 2017 Global fact sheet

5. 2011–2014 National Health and Nutrition Examination Survey (NHANES), National Center for Health Statistics, Centers for Disease Control and Prevention.

6. *Worldwide trends in blood pressure from 1975 to 2015: a pooled analysis of 1479 population-based measurement studies with 19·1 million participants*, Lancet 2017; 389: 37–55 Published Online November 15, 2016. http://dx.doi.org/10.1016/ S0140-6736(16)31919-5

7. "*Heart Disease and Stroke Statistics—2018 Update: A Report from the American Heart Association,*" Circulation (numbers rounded) Published Jan. 31, 2018

8. Mozzafarian D, Benjamin EJ, Go AS, et al. *Heart Disease and Stroke Statistics-2015 Update: a report from the American Heart Association.* Circulation. 2015;e29-322.

9. Merai R, Siegel C, Rakotz M, Basch P, Wright J, Wong B; DHSc., Thorpe P. *CDC Grand Rounds: A Public Health Approach to Detect and Control Hypertension*. MMWR Morb Mortal Wkly Rep. 2016 Nov 18;65(45):1261-1264

10. Full data on cancer deaths, including upper and lower estimates can be downloaded at the IHME's Global Burden of Disease (GBD) at http://ghdx.healthdata.org/gbd-results-tool

11. Howlader N, Noone AM, Krapcho M, Miller D, Brest A, Yu M, Ruhl J, Tatalovich Z, Mariotto A, Lewis DR, Chen HS, Feuer EJ, Cronin KA (eds). *SEER Cancer Statistics Review, 1975-2016, National Cancer Institute*. Bethesda, MD, https://seer.cancer.gov/csr/1975_2016/, based on November 2018 SEER data submission, posted to the SEER web site, April 2019.

12. American Cancer Society. *Cancer Facts & Figures 2017*. Atlanta: American Cacer Society; 2017

13. *Mapped: the global epidemic of 'lifestyle' disease in charts*, The Telegraph, Aisha Majid, global health security data journalist 29 MARCH 2018 • 3:23PM https://www.telegraph.co.uk/global-health/climate-and-people/mapped-global-epidemic-lifestyle-disease-charts/

14. *Deaths: Leading Causes for 2017*, by Melonie Heron, Ph.D., Division of Vital Statistics, National Vital Statistics Reports, Vol. 68, No. 6, June 24, 2019. https://www.cdc.gov/nchs/fastats/leading-causes-of-death.htm

15. *Egyptian Princess Mummy Had Oldest Known Heart Disease*, BY JAMES OWEN, FOR NATIONAL GEOGRAPHIC NEWS, PUBLISHED APRIL 15, 2011 https://news.nationalgeographic.com/news/2011/04/110415-ancient-egypt-mummies-princess-heart-disease-health-science/

CHAPTER 2

1. *Change Your Brain, Change Your Life: The Breakthrough Program for Conquering Anxiety, Depression, Obsessiveness, Anger, and Impulsiveness*, Dr. Daniel G. Amen, Random House, 1998

2. Wang, G-J.; Volkow, N.D.; et al. Brain dopamine and obesity. Lancet 357(9253):354-357, 2001.

3. Williamson AM, Feyer AM. Moderate sleep deprivation produces impairments in cognitive and motor performance equivalent to legally prescribed levels of alcohol intoxication. Occup Environ Med. 2000;57(10):649-55.

4. Arnedt JT, Wilde GJ, Munt PW, MacLean AW. How do prolonged wakefulness and alcohol compare in the decrements they produce on a simulated driving task? Accid Anal Prev. 2001;33(3):337-44.

5. Dawson D, Reid K. Fatigue, alcohol and performance impairment. Nature. 1997;388(6639):235.

6. Lamond N, Dawson D. Quantifying the performance impairment associated with fatigue. J Sleep Res. 1999;8(4):255-62.

CHAPTER 3

1. Brody AL, Mandelkern MA, London ED, et al. *Cigarette smoking saturates brain alpha 4 beta 2 nicotinic acetylcholine receptors*. Arch Gen Psychiatry. 2006;63(8):907–915. doi:10.1001/archpsyc.63.8.907

2. Newberg, A. B., & Waldman, M. R. (2010). *How God changes your brain: Breakthrough findings from a leading*

neuro scientist. New York: Ballantine Books Trade Paperbacks.

Visit our website at
WWW.THEWHOLELIFE.COM

www.ingramcontent.com/pod-product-compliance
Lightning Source LLC
Chambersburg PA
CBHW040823300326
41914CB00063B/1481